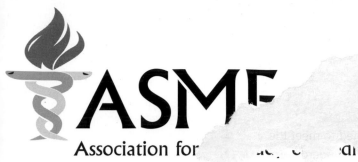

ASME
Association for

Portfolios, personal development and reflective practice

John Pitts

Understanding Medical Education

The *Understanding Medical Education* series is designed to meet the needs of all newcomers to medical education, whether undergraduate or postgraduate, including those studying at certificate, diploma and masters level. *Understanding Medical Education* aims to provide an authoritative, up-to-date and comprehensive resource summarising the theoretical and academic bases of modern medical education practice.

Publications in the series are written by experts from all walks of medical education and offer a worldwide perspective on contemporary practice. The series aims to be both accessible and useful to the reader. After reading a publication in the series the reader should not only be better informed about their field of interest, but able to assimilate their new knowledge into their clinical teaching or academic activities.

Understanding Medical Education will be published during the course of 2006–7. The full list of titles is shown below.

General

- Principles of curriculum design
- Teaching and learning in medical education: how theory can inform practice

Educational strategies

- Problem-based learning
- Inter-professional education
- Informal learning and the medical apprentice
- Learning from the humanities
- Portfolios, personal development and reflective practice

Educational encounters

- Supervision, mentoring and coaching
- Teaching and leading small groups
- Lectures and large groups
- eLearning
- Simulation in medical education

Assessment

- How to design a useful test
- Written examinations
- Workplace-based assessment in clinical training
- Assessment of clinical competence
- Formative assessment
- Self-assessment

Research and evaluation

- Thinking about research: frameworks, ethics and scholarship
- Quantitative research methods in medical education
- Qualitative research methods in medical education
- Evaluation: improving education, influencing policy

Staff and students

- Best practice selection for medical education and training
- Identifying poor performance and managing remediation
- Quality in medical education
- Dealing with diversity
- The development of medical educators
- Educational leadership

Icons

Throughout the *Understanding Medical Education* series readers will come across a number of icons in the margin. These graphic devices serve to highlight certain insert boxes where the author wishes to take the reader off into a particular area in greater detail (⚗ Focus on), explore the evidence behind a particular concept (🖊 Where's the evidence), provide practical advice (👈 How to) or summarise the main points of the paper (🔒 Key messages).

Contents

Introduction   1

Contents of a portfolio   1

Purposes of portfolios in medicine and nursing   3

    Continuing professional development   4

    Enhanced learning   5

    Assessment   6

    Evaluation   7

    Certification and re-certification   8

    Career advancement   8

Assessment through portfolios   10

    Philosophical issues behind assessment   10

Reflective practice and professional development   12

    Reflective practice   12

    Personal development in professional life   14

    Professional knowledge   15

    Professional practice   15

An interpretive approach to portfolio assessment   16

Conclusions   17

Acknowledgement   18

References   19

Further reading   24

Author: John Pitts

John Pitts MSc (Med Ed) PhD MRCP FRCGP is Associate Director in Educational Research, NHS (Severn & Wessex Deanery), Honorary Research Fellow at the University of Winchester and editor of the journal *Education for Primary Care*.

Editor: Tim Swanwick

The *Understanding Medical Education* series has been brought together and edited by Dr Tim Swanwick. Tim has a broad range of experience in general practice education and educational leadership. Currently a Director of Postgraduate General Practice Education in the London Deanery and an Honorary Senior Lecturer at Imperial College, Tim is the editor of *Understanding Medical Education*, sits on the editorial board of the journal *Education for Primary Care*, and writes widely on all aspects of GP education and training. He is co-author of *The Study Guide for GP Training* (2003), and editor of *The General Practice Journey* (2003) and *The Management Handbook for Primary Care* (2004).

Production of such a major series is a team effort and thanks must go to the *Understanding Medical Education* advisory board for their editorial guidance, Jill Cropper for her expert copy editing, Brian Cairns at the publishing house Blue Square, and Nicky Pender and the ASME team for their unfailing and efficient administrative support.

Views expressed in this publication are necessarily those of the author(s) and should not be construed as official ASME policy.

Key messages:

- Resistance to the idea of a portfolio from learners, teachers and managers should be seen and understood within the prevailing culture.

- Portfolio-based learning has the potential to explore and develop an individual's professional practice.

- Portfolios embrace the professional artistry model of professional practice.

- Traditional approaches to assessment may be inappropriate for portfolios. In portfolio assessment, validity is more important than reliability and the reliability may be supplanted by the qualitative concept of trustworthiness.

- The expert judgement of the teacher will always be part of the assessment process, hence teacher development is essential.

- When assessment is used for regulatory high-stakes purposes, it should follow on from the formative processes that have enabled the professional to learn.

- Portfolios can be used as an acceptable and understandable method of professional accreditation and re-accreditation if traditional views and prejudices are set aside.

Introduction

Rooted in the principles of experiential learning, portfolio-based learning is an approach that has the 'critical intellectual task of moving from a description of an experience to the identification of the learning derived from that experience and ultimately deciding what further education is required to fill in gaps revealed by the analysis of the described experience. It recognises the value and significance of past learning and experience for the individual; the ability of adults to learn and act autonomously; the centrality of reflection in the learning process and the need for meaningful links to be made between experiences, learning opportunities and role requirements'.[1]

Although there may be many differences in purpose, structure and assessment requirements, certain key aspects are usually highlighted:

- the *experience* – what has happened, what has been done, seen, written, made, etc.

- the *learning* – the discovery that what has been recalled has significance for doing or changing things in the future

- the *evidence* – a demonstration of how the learning is being applied in a particular context

- *learning needs* – an identification of where it would be appropriate to go next

- *learning opportunities* – an educational action plan identifying ways in which learning needs might be met.[2]

A major characteristic is that the learner selects the contents, which may include a curriculum vitae, log books, case reports, critical incidents[3] and significant event auditing,[4] clinical data, written evaluations, audits, research projects, accounts of innovations, critical reading exercises and videotapes of performance. But it is important that the structure is not too rigid; a portfolio is a means to an end, not an end in itself.

Throughout the rest of this paper, the use of portfolios in medical education will be discussed under the three broad and interrelated headings of **contents**, **purposes** and **assessment**.

Contents of a portfolio

The first challenge is to define what a portfolio is, or is not. At its widest, the term has been used to include course logs, dossiers, logbooks, training records and folders, and does not necessarily include the benefits and processes listed above. Such documents may exclude any evidence of reflection and self-analysis, and this has led to confusion in the understanding and evaluation of the portfolio approach.[5] Established definitions more clearly include those elements. For example, 'a purposeful collection of student work that exhibits the student's efforts, progress and achievements in one or more areas. The collection must include student participation in selecting contents, the criteria for selection, the criteria for judging merit and evidence of self-reflection'.[6]

Further definitions are: 'a collection of evidence which demonstrates the continuing acquisition of knowledge, skills, attitudes, understanding and achievements … reflecting the current stages of development and activity of the individual'[7]; and 'a professional development portfolio is a collection of material, made by a professional, that records and reflects on key events and processes in that professional's career'.[8] The latter definition is particularly noteworthy because of the inclusion of the term 'professional'.

In terms of how material is collected and collated, Webb and colleagues[9] outlined four portfolio models in common use. Each model structures the content in a different way. The four types are highlighted in Box 1.

 BOX 1 **Models of portfolios[9]**

Shopping trolley

The portfolio is used to collect anything that could be seen as a vehicle to learning and the choice is limited only by what the student considers to be appropriate. There are rarely any linking strategies between components.

Toast rack

The portfolio contains a number of pre-determined 'slots' that must be filled for each module of a programme, e.g. action plans, reflective accounts of significant events, skills checklists. Each component is formally assessed in isolation.

Cake mix

The parts of the portfolio are blended in that students are expected to provide evidence that they have achieved specified learning outcomes while on placement. The 'mixing' is provided by reflective commentaries addressing analytical criteria.

Spinal column

A series of competency statements form the central column of the portfolio and students collect evidence to demonstrate their achievement. One piece of evidence may be used against multiple statements.

Currently, the majority of portfolios in existence are paper-based, although audio-taped and videotaped material may be included where appropriate. Many organisations have developed 'off-the-shelf' portfolio formats, and there is a large growth in the use of electronic formats in both postgraduate and undergraduate medical education.[10–13] E-portfolios differ from paper-based ones in that there is generally a higher level of standardisation, and issues of mentoring and support and assessment processes present a challenge. In theory, it is possible for the contents of an e-portfolio to include video recordings and online assessments, so technological developments will offer increasing depth and scope. However, e-learning in this way does not appeal to everyone – a small-scale evaluation in UK primary care showed that only a minority completed what they had signed up for[14] – and careful implementation and training are, as with all portfolio-based approaches, vital.

It is clear that the contents of a portfolio can vary greatly, both in terms of the material within, and from prescriptive to 'free range'. An important distinction can be made between inclusions that are *indirect*, i.e. information *about* the writer, and *direct*, i.e. created *by* the writer. This allows, for example, for the inclusion of performance data such as audit results *and* reflections and conclusions thereon.

Content, however, is ultimately dictated by purpose.

Purposes of portfolios in medicine and nursing

There must be a clear reason for the existence of a portfolio. Some are used to record personal development and career progression, while others may be assessed for specific purposes such as the demonstration of a certain level of achievement. They range from personal documents held in privacy to a high-stakes assessment approach such as a 'final' examination.[15] Tomkinson[16] (Box 2) suggested a taxonomy for the development of portfolios where each characteristic represents a point at either end of a continuum. Discussions between all parties involved about where on this continuum a portfolio should be situated can make explicit how and what should be achieved and expressed.

BOX 2 **A taxonomy for the development of portfolios[16]**

Dimension of portfolio design	Possible characteristics	
Style	Descriptive	Reflective
Structure	Informal	Formal
Scope	Narrow (e.g. teaching activity)	Broad (e.g. all clinical and non-clinical activities)
Purpose	Developmental (formative)	Assessment (summative)
Confidentiality	Personal (closed)	Public (open)
Content	Focused (e.g. critical incidents)	Comprehensive (e.g. range of contexts and data)
Timing	Discrete	Continuous

Within the published literature, six distinct, sometimes overlapping yet complementary, purposes can be identified (Box 3). We will explore these further.

BOX 3   Uses of portfolios

- Continuing professional development
- Enhanced learning
- Assessment
- Evaluation
- Certification and re-certification
- Career advancement

Continuing professional development

A substantial part of published literature refers to the use of portfolios in recording and demonstrating an individual's continuing professional development. In one study in UK nursing, an integrated system of professional development was established between an NHS trust hospital and a school of nursing and midwifery. This aimed to build a model of clinical supervision which developed standards for clinical competence that facilitated continuity in professional development throughout the practitioner's career. The collaboration between the two organisations ensured that the model reflected links between theory and practice, and encompassed the requirements of the UK Central Council for Nursing (UKCC) and the English National Board for Nursing, Midwifery and Health Visiting (ENB).[17]

In the United States, teaching portfolios for nurse educators have been used for both formative and summative purposes, and have been described as an effective solution to the dilemma of 'how to comprehensively present oneself as a teacher' (sic).[18] Building on this, two principal purposes for teaching portfolios were identified:

- to assist in the growth and development of the teacher
- to document teaching effectiveness for personnel reasons such as promotion and tenure.[19]

In medicine, a working party of the Royal College of General Practitioners[1] advocated a portfolio-based approach for continuing professional development for general practitioners. Following this, an autonomous learning project for a group of GPs, using the support of mentors, was piloted and found to be both acceptable and assessable through a checklist of quality of evidence,[20] an approach also used successfully with a group of newly established GPs attending a higher professional education course.[21] In general practice vocational training, groups of general practice registrars found portfolios to be of value in reminding, planning, tracking and encouraging reflection; as a route to exploring attitudes and values to stimulate feedback; as encouragement, not humiliation; and to act as a bridge from hospital practice to general practice.[22,23] As a means of recording continuing professional development for a group of GPs, completed portfolios were judged against efficiency (effort expended) and effectiveness (distance travelled), and satisfactory completion accredited for the postgraduate education allowance.[24] In a review of continuing professional development for GPs by the Chief Medical Officer in England, a practice-based portfolio – the practice professional development plan – was proposed[25] and broadly welcomed.[26] A project in Wales explored the potential for portfolios to enhance the learning of a group of GPs through 'professional dialogues'. Evaluation showed that there was strong support for portfolio-based learning; participants felt that their learning was very valuable, and attributed this in large part to the effect of the group.[27]

An evaluation of the use of an electronic portfolio for continuing professional development of consultant physicians in the UK demonstrated a high level of support in principle, although resource shortages limited its use.[28]

Enhanced learning

Another reason for using portfolios is to improve the effectiveness of learning. The use of portfolios as a strategy to support learner-centred learning in student nurses has also been studied.[29] Incorporating reflection on prior experiences, forward planning to meet course outcomes, critical incident analysis and a reflective journal, the portfolio was described as 'an attempt to enable the different knowledge bases of theory and practice to be bridged'. Its greatest gain was in the way the students moved from teacher dependency to self-direction. Presenting teaching accomplishments through a portfolio promoted self-reflection and a direction for improvement and advancement decisions.[30] At the start of the process, nurse educators felt lack of motivation, uncertainty as to what was expected, and anxiety about sharing personal thoughts and feelings. Peer assessment provided another source of concern, although the activity was ultimately seen as a positive experience, with both faculty and peer observers reporting having gained insight into each others' teaching practice and styles. After a situational analysis demonstrated a need for planned learning in an orthopaedic/trauma unit, an action research project explored whether portfolio preparation was itself developmental and if so, what factors influenced this.[31] The findings suggested that the process itself influenced development by acting as an initiator to reflection on experience.

In medicine, the educational effectiveness of prolonged community-based attachments for undergraduate medical students has been assessed using portfolios. Popular with both tutors and students, the educational achievements were rated as satisfactory or outstanding.[32] Reflective portfolios supported by a mentoring process have been used with success in Holland with undergraduate medical students.[33] In a group of registrars in general practice training, a portfolio-based approach worked well for some, but not all.[22] For those in favour, the portfolio became an important means of capturing the events of the training year to reflect on progress made and to define and set future learning needs. The authors concluded that in addition, this approach required considerable support and encouragement from the general practice trainers responsible for the registrars. Similarly, in an interview study, reflective practice was claimed as an outcome of a course for medical educators.[34]

Portfolios have a good level of acceptance as vehicles for providing evidence of continuing professional development as a means of privately and publicly demonstrating professional growth, and documenting professional effectiveness.

However, for senior house officers in accident and emergency departments and an obstetric unit, using personal learning logs in the format of a controlled study did not increase learning in the study group.[35] The authors commented that the contents of the logs revealed great scope for learning, but few doctors documented the specific learning achieved, and that for the initiative to be successful, active participation from trained senior staff, protected time for learning and a 'more positive approach from all concerned' would be needed.

The use of an electronic portfolio using a personal computer-based software program showed that users who agreed with the statement 'entering items of learning into my diary encourages me to think in terms of questions that guide my learning' recorded an attempt 'to modify their practice' as an outcome more often than those who disagreed with that statement.[36] An examination of the portfolios of medical teachers for 'reflectiveness' found good evidence,[37] yet concluded that set assignments could be too directive.[38]

Assessment

Formative assessment

Formative assessment, through feedback from teachers or peers, is a major benefit of portfolio learning. By providing the opportunity to review and reflect on progress, and through this, to reset objectives and goals, it is possible to monitor and shape learning. Beyond factual learning and recorded experience, reflection on issues behind events and situations allows and encourages the exploration and expression of assumptions, beliefs and values that underpin such experiences. Much of the published literature alludes to this, although details are sparse. The willingness of writers to commit to deeper expression is likely to be related to knowledge and trust of the mentor or supervisor.

In a study of undergraduates training in obstetrics and gynaecology, a structured portfolio was used to record practical procedures carried out and the individual reflections of students.[39] Group sessions tutored by consultants were also used as the basis for further reflections and the identification of future learning. The authors concluded that portfolios supported the development of complex skills, clarified learning goals and helped students to monitor their achievement. Currently in the UK, continuing educational requirements for pre-registration house officers[40] and the Record of In-service Training Assessments (RITAs) for specialist registrars[41] are met through a similar portfolio approach.

The value of a portfolio approach in formative assessment is probably the least contentious application, because it is individually related, developmental and does not have to address the murky issue of robust judgement.

Summative assessment

The use of portfolios in summative assessment is still relatively untested. This is because of difficulties in addressing the issue of reliability, which is held as vitally important from the perspective of traditional assessment methodology and the prevailing positivist viewpoint, and the demonstration of a high level of 'trustworthiness' if a non-positivist viewpoint is taken. Generally speaking, portfolios have high face validity, but there are problems with reliability, relating to both content specificity and rater issues,[42,43] and deep suspicion in relation to the role of self-assessment.[44,45]

Portfolios encourage reflectiveness, empower a learner-centred approach to learning, allow self-assessment, and provide the ability to record and fulfil future learning needs. Personal commitment, motivation, shared values, senior and institutional support are important predictors of success.

The medical school at the University of Dundee uses portfolio assessment in the final year examinations of medical students.[15] Evaluation of the first year of this process revealed strong support from staff and generally positive reactions from the students. The contents included clinical case reports and reflections thereon, practical procedure records, needs-based learning agreements, special study module assessment forms and reports, reports of an elective activity and a fourth-year assignment report. The assessment process comprised an initial grading followed by a session where four examiners (three internal, one external), working in pairs, reviewed each portfolio with the student. Conclusions from the evaluation were that portfolio building provided a bridge between formative and summative assessment, and a means of monitoring the progress of students. While concluding that portfolio assessment is a useful tool that provides a powerful approach to assessing a range of curricular outcomes not easily assessed by other methods, and may even provide a basis for a judgement on 'fitness to practise', there is a comment that 'attention must be paid to logistics with careful briefing of examiners and students'.

Using a checklist approach based on the five criteria of logical and coherent structure, level of critical reflection, level of actual or future skills development, use of documentary evidence and use of relevant literature, a summative assessment process for medical students produced a reliability of overall scores of 0.77 when two assessors jointly rated the portfolios,[46] thereby matching the 'best' objective tests. However, to reach similar levels of reliability in assessing GPs' learning plans, it has been calculated that five to eight assessors are required.[47] More recently, portfolios have been used successfully in the summative assessment of medical students at the University of Maastricht,[48] and here a purely qualitative methodology has been adopted, with the concept of *reliability* replaced with that of *trustworthiness*, a key issue in portfolio assessment that we will consider in more detail later.

Evaluation

Portfolios completed by learners offer an opportunity to judge the effects and effectiveness of the teaching and learning. In nursing, student nurse portfolios have been used to evaluate undergraduate nursing programmes. Portfolios represent a more realistic appraisal of what students are learning and allow validation of programme outcomes for both the institution and external agencies, as well as certification of competency. They also ensure that teachers know that their efforts have been effective and that intended learning has occurred. Overall, portfolios were seen as an opportunity to showcase a variety of work to demonstrate the attainment of professional competence and increase faculty–student collaboration and shared learning.[49]

In some fields of medicine, the gathering of evidence of 'quality of teaching' in the form of a teacher's portfolio has been used.[50] The implementation of teaching portfolios for clinical teachers, while showing strong support from the academic leadership, revealed extraordinary pressures on staff to minimise engagement in teaching, an insufficient infrastructure to support documentation of educational quality, and conflicts between an external economic reward system and the valuing of teaching.[51] These authors concluded that there are significant challenges to those who chose academic medicine for its educational focus, and those who desired recognition and validation of those activities.

There is great potential for portfolios as a tool for summative assessment, because of the nature of professional learning and professional practice, and also because of the deficiencies of existing assessment methods.

A log diary approach that encouraged medical students in internal medicine and community-based clerkship to record activities with patients and their teachers recorded both the use of time and the perceived quality of their teaching,[52] and a portfolio learning approach was used to provide individual evaluation of the teachers.[39]

Certification and re-certification

In many ways the same issues that confound and confuse portfolio use in summative assessments are relevant here. In any high-stakes assessment that can affect a person's livelihood and remuneration, there must be a high degree of trust that any judgement made is the 'right one'.

The UK Central Council for Nursing (UKCC)[53] requires nurses 'to effectively demonstrate (sic) that they have taken action to maintain and develop professional knowledge and competence … to use a personal professional profile'. The English National Board for Nursing, Midwifery and Health Visiting (ENB)[54] similarly sees a professional portfolio as 'an essential part of the board's framework for continuing professional education'. Commenting on this, Jasper[55] stated that portfolio compilation had great potential provided that attempts were made to ensure its relevance to the practitioner and that a solid infrastructure of educational, managerial and financial support was in place.

In medicine in the United Kingdom, in order to fulfil the requirements of both annual appraisal and revalidation, all doctors are expected to maintain a 'folder' that includes an educational record, performance data, audit and evidence of effective communication with patients. These portfolios are structured according to areas defined by the General Medical Council in its publication *Good Medical Practice*.[56] These include: good clinical care, maintaining good medical practice, relationships with patients, working with colleagues, teaching and training, research, probity and health.

Career advancement

Using a peer-reviewed portfolio as a basis for promotion in nursing has been described, where criteria that identify functioning as a role model, teaching colleagues and introducing change are used in a process of assessment by peer review.[57] Promotions via this 'clinical ladder system' were also accompanied by increases in salary. A summative evaluation of a baccalaureate programme for nurse development demonstrated that a portfolio approach represented a positive option for career development.[58] This was shown to reflect adult learning theory and provide maximum opportunity and flexibility for students to meet the leadership and management requirements of the course. The notion of a portfolio-based presentation at an annual appraisal as a means of moving away from the narrow areas of teaching, research and service towards the broader creative and reflective activities of the professional has been promoted,[18] and the potential for teaching portfolios as a means of provision of documentation for promotion and tenure purposes has also been identified.[19]

In the US, documentation of teaching accomplishments related to established criteria of effective teaching behaviour has been incorporated into a teaching portfolio and used in promotion, tenure and salary decisions about clinical medical staff. Beyond this, the university used the perceived quality of

Portfolios provide an opportunity for teachers to both assess themselves and receive feedback on their activities from their learners. Institutional support and commitment are prerequisites for success.

Portfolios can provide a longitudinal record of a career, presenting evidence of professional attributes and activities for external scrutiny.

educational activity by means of the educators' portfolios to decide the distribution of funds between departments.[50] A survey of 134 medical schools in the US in 1994[59] revealed that 20% had a portfolio system in place, 8% were in the process of developing one and 21% were in discussion about it. Of those currently using this approach, the prime purpose was for supporting decisions of career promotion. A survey of all the medical schools in the US plus those in Canada three years later, showed that about half had a 'clinician-educator promotion track' based on an evaluation strategy that used a combination of awards, peer evaluations, learner evaluations and teaching portfolios. This formed the basis of promotion decisions for the majority of schools.[60]

The use of a portfolio throughout a career is becoming established as an accepted means of providing evidence for career advancement.

BOX 4   Where's the evidence? Themes from the literature

- There is growth in portfolio usage in healthcare education despite reservations and shortcomings.

- Portfolio users gain from the experience in their learning, understanding, concepts of 'empowerment' as adult learners and control over their learning, and in relationships with their teachers and tutors.

- The ability of portfolios to provide documentary evidence to demonstrate proficiency is held as a major strength.

- Benefits go beyond individuals. Teachers, departments and institutions all gain from the process and information gathered.

- In high-stakes assessment, reliability is seen as a problem, but rigour may be established through the adoption of qualitative paradigms.

- Users in all studies report preconceptions of difficulty, uncertainty in what was expected and a lack of confidence in their ability to build the required portfolio.

Focus on: Acceptability

A recurring theme when portfolios are introduced is uncertainty and confusion, followed by acceptance and understanding of value. Participants' responses to a reflective portfolio-based learning approach have been classified into hierarchical models. In a study of the developmental processes through which training experiences are elaborated and professional identity gained, pre-clinical medical students' approaches to professional self-reflection and identity formation could be defined as: 'committed reflection', 'emotional exploration', 'objective reporting' and 'diffuse reporting'.[61]

Similarly, GPs using a 'personal professional journal' to reflect on day-to-day work were classified as 'descriptive', 'analytical' or 'evaluative'.[62]

These findings indicate that the usefulness of a portfolio to the learning process may vary with the type of project and the stage that the learner has reached in developing the particular practical wisdom associated with the practice of medicine. This will grow as a result of experience and the amount they are helped to see the wisdom behind their judgements through reflection and deliberation. Reflective portfolios may be of limited use in the early stages of learning when the learner does not know enough about the subject, or lacks appropriate experience to raise relevant questions, but they can provide a vehicle through which authentic experience can be used as a basis for reflection and professional development. In other words, there is a maturity of response through which confidence grows, and this must be taken into account when the introduction and assessment of portfolios is considered.

Assessment through portfolios

As an assessment instrument, portfolios have particular advantages, primarily stemming from the differences between a portfolio and a 'typical' examination situation, which is a pressurised and stressful time-limited event occurring at the end of a course or programme. Portfolios are not, intrinsically, an examination method, yet they can be used as a basis for assessment. Completing the portfolio over time allows for multiple attempts and opportunities, revision and reflection, and it can address multiple tasks and use many forms of data entry. Furthermore, portfolios offer the chance to continue to be both a record of personal development and a career log. They may be seen as an *authentic* assessment – one that looks at performance and practical application of theory.[23,63] The principal disadvantages stem from unfamiliarity, the effort involved and, in terms of assessment, the lack of evidence for supporting judgements that may be made.

Philosophical issues behind assessment

A fundamental issue with this relatively new (to medicine) approach to learning as an assessment method is the difficulty in making it fit with traditional views of an assessment process.[64] The paradox is that developing this to its full potential moves away from objective and standardised testing towards a subjective and non-standardised position.[65] To achieve high reliability means sacrificing individuality by constricting and controlling the format, and scoring according to some template or checklist. This thereby limits the greatest value of a portfolio to the individual, which is as a reflective tool – a personal account of professional practice that identifies and acknowledges both strengths and weaknesses. However, some authors have argued that in non-standardised assessments, reliability becomes less important.[48,66] In this area, it should be borne in mind that for many years there seems to have been little difficulty with the summative judgement of dissertations, theses, etc., or the selection of material for publication. Furthermore, much published work on portfolio assessment uses statistical methodology to assess inter-rater reliability that is inconsistent and open to challenge.[42] Kappa statistics are the most appropriate since they take into account chance agreement, they can be adapted to different numbers of assessors, different assessors can be used for different portfolios and different numbers of assessors can be used for each portfolio.[67] Introducing the notion of external assessment alters learners' approaches to learning, which becomes directed towards the perceived purposes of the examination strategy.[68] How is this likely to influence what goes into a portfolio? Surely it will not be thought that identifying and displaying weaknesses will impress an examiner? Although perhaps now less rigidly interpreted than earlier, it may be that traditional psychometric views of reliability and validity are limiting more meaningful educational approaches.

Assessment approaches that attempt to measure the learning processes shown by portfolios require a different set of educational values that recognise the role of personal and professional judgements on the part of the learner. Reflective behaviour involves the practitioner investigating and seeking insights into their practice. It accepts the subjectivity of data and interpretations, and focuses on individual insights and development. It values creativity and, importantly, allows and understands the possibility of being wrong. Phillips[69] quoted Thomas Kuhn, who popularised the notion that inquirers always work within a paradigm or framework that determines the concepts that are used. He stated that in a sense, all inquirers are trapped within their own paradigms; they will judge certain things as being true (for them) that others will judge as being false (for them). This highlights the issue that assessors and their subjects carry, perhaps unwittingly, personal agendas into the assessment process that can lead to undue weightings and bias. Open discussions may go some way to improve reliability by making explicit the otherwise unstated assumptions, beliefs and values of the assessors.[70] While in general, standardisation and structuring of assessment may improve reliability,[71] this may explain why traditionally high levels are not easily reached.

To explore this impasse, we need to consider the nature of reflective practice and what it means to practise as a professional.

Reflective practice and professional development

Reflective practice

The term 'reflective practice' first appears in the work of Dewey,[72] and was expanded on in the 1980s by authors such as Schön.[73] Reflective practice has been defined as: 'the process of internally examining and exploring an issue of concern, triggered by an experience, which creates and clarifies meaning in terms of self, and which results in a changed conceptual perspective'.[74] Schön[75] made a distinction between reflection-in-action and reflection-on-action, where the former is represented by 'questioning the assumptional structures of knowing-in-action' and thinking critically about 'the thinking that got us into this fix or this opportunity'.

Practical experience is at the centre of professional learning,[76] and it has been suggested that educational programmes should include reflective processes based on personal experiences.[77] Learning is the process of transforming experiences into knowledge, skills, attitudes and values, and as such has been represented graphically by means of experiential/learning cycles, for example that of Kolb (Figure 1).[78]

Figure 1 Kolb's cycle of experiential learning.[78]

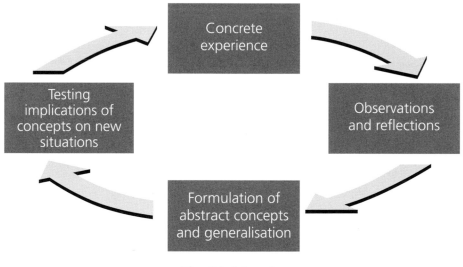

The 'Kolb' cycle

Concrete experience, observations and reflections, formulation of abstract concepts and generalisations, and the testing of implications of concepts in new situations are the stations around this cyclical model. Jarvis[79] believed this to be oversimplistic, and developed a model that represents a more complex model of learning, suggesting nine possible responses to an experience, divisible into three categories, which include non-learning and non-reflective learning as well as reflective learning. Non-learning included responses such as: presumption, where previous learned experiences are trusted and comfortably taken for granted; non-consideration, where people are too busy or uncomfortable to explore further; and rejection, where the possibility of learning from an experience is rejected, sometimes, for example, through bias or bigotry. Non-reflective learning includes pre-conscious or incidental learning, the learning of repetitive or mechanical skills and memorisation. These might be detected when a portfolio is discussed through mentoring or an assessment process.

Most literature on experiential learning refers to learning from primary events, which are subjectively experienced. It is important to consider, and value, learning from secondary experiences of others, communicated in writing or verbally, by individuals or within groups. Within professions, such interactions within the community of practice represent a powerful means of learning not just about factual knowledge but about values, truths and meaning. This supports the inclusion of indirect data within a portfolio for reflection.

Sparks-Langer and Colton[80] suggested that there are three elements within reflection: cognition, critical thinking and narrative enquiry. Schön referred to these processes as *problem setting*, and believed that professional learning stems from continuous action and reflection on everyday problems. Such knowledge is often tacit and difficult to identify and analyse. Knowledge is constructed; as a professional reflects on an experience, they develop their own theoretical system. Ross[81] identified a series of steps in reflective thinking:

- recognising the nature of the problem

- responding by recognising similarities and differences to other consequences and implications of possible solution

- examining the intended and unintended consequences of the solution selected.

A similar approach is illustrated in Box 6.

BOX 6   Reflective practice – A model

A situation with no ready response:

- What was the nature of the problem?

- What were the consequences?

- How was it addressed?

- What was learned about (a) the problem and (b) myself?

- How will the same or a similar situation be addressed next time?

A key theme in reflection is an emphasis on a natural approach, where, in contrast to experiments and studies that control variables and aim for generalisable results, emphasis is given to meanings and interpretations to gain insights into practice and an appreciation of its complexity.

It is clear, therefore, that reflection is not a form of armchair relaxation best carried out alone. Assisting reflection by using colleagues, mentors and small groups, and writing down for preservation and future use, are valuable strategies that can be called upon. By reflecting on and theorising their practice, practitioners can make public, and therefore open to scrutiny and assessment, their processes of professional development.

Personal development in professional life

Learning in professional life, in the day-to-day reality of a professional's actual working practices, most importantly involves learning through reflection and conversations with peers. This establishes the important notion of a 'community of practice', a concept that will be discussed in more detail later. While there is potential for learning in any situation, the greatest source of learning is from other human beings, in particular peers and patients. Conversations around the interesting or unusual case, the problem shared that leads to the 'why don't you try...' form the very basis of peer group learning.

An increasing body of research has explored the situated character of human understanding and communication and examined the relationship between learning and the social situation in which it occurs,[82] regarding learning as a form of social co-participation, rather than the mere acquisition of knowledge. Conventional explanations see learning as the internalisation of knowledge, however acquired, leaving the nature of the learner, the world and its inter-relationships outside and unconsidered. Situated learning has two perspectives.[83] The first implies an interactive and productive role for the skills acquired – the learner is not gaining a corpus of knowledge to be used at some later time, rather the skills to perform by actually engaging in the process under the modified conditions of *legitimate peripheral participation*.[82] This allows the learner to participate in the practice of an expert professional, but in a way limited by degree and responsibility. This term provides a way to speak about relationships, between newcomers and established practitioners, and activities and communities of practice. The process of joining to become a full participant is a sociocultural process that subsumes the learning of knowledgeable skills.

The second perspective, in contrast to the view that learning occurs within the individual, is that learning takes place in a framework of participation, mediated by differences in perspective of the co-participants. It is the 'community' that learns. Whereas the learner, as an apprentice, may learn most, others learn as co-learners. The apprentices, therefore, cause changes in the larger community of practitioners. The community of practice itself contains a wide range of players, including, in addition to apprentices, young masters with apprentices themselves, as well as established practitioners who may be reaching the end of their careers. Interestingly, to sustain collaborative participation there must be conflicts between the forces that support the process of learning and those that oppose them. Within a professional group, this implies a collective grouping such as a professional organisation or trade union that stands up for the values and status of the group against what are perceived as external threats.

Learning in clinical practice moves through the stage of the novice, perhaps the medical student who 'observes', towards a notion of supervised practice, perhaps the junior doctor, who can call on a more senior member of staff if they are uncertain about how to proceed with a problem that is felt to be beyond their capability. Consequent learning is located in the increasing access of the learner to participatory roles in expert practice.[82] Even for established professionals, groups learn together through an often asymmetric co-participation in practice. Clinical practice is littered with tales told in conversations about difficulties and disasters, i.e. significant events,[4] which can lead to reconsideration of practice, reflection and adaptive learning by the wider audience.

Even for established professionals, groups learn together through an often asymmetric co-participation in practice. Clinical practice is littered with tales told in conversations about difficulties and disasters ... which can lead to reconsideration of practice, reflection and adaptive learning by the wider audience.

After a review of portfolio usage, an 'integrated proficiency-criterion framework' that linked levels of proficiency was proposed (novice, advanced beginner, competent), with outcome criteria in areas such as critical thinking, communication skills, therapeutic interventions, professional development, personal development and scholarship, allowing an assessment of an individual's overall competence.[84] This suggests that a process of maturation can be captured by means of a portfolio approach.

Professional knowledge

More light can be cast on the debate by considering the complex nature of professional knowledge. Eraut[85] divided professional knowledge into propositional, personal and process knowledge. While propositional knowledge resides in the public domain and is discipline based, personal knowledge is individually acquired by experience. Process knowledge is represented as knowing how to conduct the various processes that contribute to professional action, including knowing how to access and use propositional knowledge.[85] Schön[75] refers to many areas of professional practice as 'messy confusing problems that deny technical solution'. These may be best explored through a reflective approach. Among the implications for professional education and assessment are conclusions that are in direct opposition to the existing systems, as in reality any assessment of professional competence that fails to observe in some way the hidden aspect of one's expertise cannot be held to be valid.[86]

Schön[75] refers to many areas of professional practice as 'messy confusing problems that deny technical solution.

Professional practice

A further angle on the issue of assessment may be gained by considering the two models of professional practice described by Fish.[87] The first is the *technical-rational model*, which assumes that professional activity is a matter of technical performance, following a logical sequence as part of an efficient system. This values the technical aspects of the professional's work (measurable skills, performance and procedures that can be mastered) and logical systems and efficiency. This behavioural model assumes that professional activity consists of actions that are visible, observable and therefore amenable to measurement. The emphasis is on pre-determined skills and procedures, and permanent and quantifiable propositional knowledge, and the process of measurement strives for objectivity. Fish argues that technical accountability has to be controlled by elaborate mechanisms of assessment, inspection, appraisal and accreditation, beneath which lies the view that professionals are not to be trusted – in other words, not fit to exercise professional judgement.

A second, alternative, view is the *professional artistry model*, which sees professional practice as an art. It stresses understanding rather than technical skills, and takes a holistic approach to skills and knowledge. Within a core knowledge of skills and routines it accepts that it is not possible to know everything, and sees open capacities and competencies that cannot be mastered as more valuable than closed ones that can, but are usually more trivial.[88] This model stresses investigation and reflection on practice, with the practitioner investigating and seeking insights into their practice. It accepts the essential subjectivity of data and any interpretations made, and focuses on individual insights and development. It accepts professional behaviour as self-regulating; beneath this model lies a view of professionals as deserving certain autonomy as a result of knowledge and moral responsibility. Its view about defining standards is that what is below standard is perfectly easily recognised when seen. There is no need for a complex 'schedule' of basic competence (which, unless very basic, will not be agreed upon by assessors), as it cannot take account of the unique practitioner in a unique practice.

An interpretive approach to portfolio assessment

If we accept the notion that portfolios are individual and subjective, how might an assessment process look? An assessor would need to see that the work within a portfolio is *valid*, showing what it claims to show, and *sufficient*, detailed enough for an assessor to infer that learning has indeed taken place.[89] Along with the need for the work done to have been sufficiently recent, i.e. *current*, to be meaningful, these constitute the degree of *authenticity* of the portfolio. The portfolio can be 'placed' in context on the continuum contained within a taxonomy of characteristics such as that of Tomkinson,[12] through discussions between the assessed and the assessors. This means that the purpose of the assessment is defined, overt and understood, and can be seen in relationship to where the learner is starting from and, at some point of judgement, how far the learner has travelled. Having ascertained the purpose, the choice of and responsibility for the contents can be devolved to the learner. This offers the opportunity for the individual, metaphorically, to talk about their practice and explore the beliefs and values involved. The source of evidence should be indicated; some will be direct (i.e. created by the learner), such as reflective accounts and audits, and some will be indirect (i.e. about the learner), such as performance statistics and correspondence. During the construction of the portfolio, collaboration with at least one other person will enhance development and provide feedback through assisted reflection and discussion.[90] Similarly, at the point at which an external judgement is required, discussions with and between the assessors allow opportunities for explanation, clarification and context setting. Merely taking part in the process is not sufficient. Assessors are, regardless of and independently of others, able to identify features that they take to be 'good practice' and areas with which they take issue. Discussion between two assessors, and perhaps also the writer of the portfolio, can enhance understanding and meaning such that the assessors can judge whether the writer is doing satisfactorily and exhibiting appropriate qualities and behaviours or, conversely, is not showing the learning and insights that they perhaps could. As a living instrument, the work in question can be revisited, reviewed, reconsidered, rewritten and resubmitted in the light of that conversation.

Over a predetermined period of time, learning needs identified can be recorded and incorporated into a 'learning contract'.[91,92] At subsequent review, fulfilment and completion of an agreement can be included within the assessment process.

Such a truly authentic approach would allow an individual's continuing professional development to be followed, encouraged and understood, perhaps over some considerable period of time, and values improvements made above deficiencies highlighted. Furthermore, a portfolio process avoids the philosophical trap of the 'false dualism' that forces one assessment approach to be taken to the exclusion of another. Taking a quantitative approach where appropriate, for example for aspects of professional practice that are generalisable, and a qualitative one in areas that are individual avoids this and places portfolio assessment within a model that focuses on the professional's progress as a developmental ideal.

> ### BOX 7   How to: Introduce a portfolio, successfully
>
> - Be clear about the purpose of the portfolio
> - In design, consider together content, purpose and assessment
> - Understand the level of experience and maturity of the learner
> - Maintain the centrality of 'reflection on practice'
> - Base on individual professional practice
> - Provide clear instructions for use
> - Develop and implement a well-resourced training strategy
> - Provide institutional support and leadership

Conclusions

The portfolio approach has many advantages, both theoretical and practical. At the beginning it allows individuals to define who and where they are, to take stock of their professional positions. Following reflective cycles of learning, disassembling and critically reconstructing their practice, drawing conclusions and planning learning are all in accord with theories of effective learning. The approach is congruent with the nature of professional knowledge, practice and how professionals learn, and represents a means of capturing the exercising of professional judgement. The process of writing represents a form of 'conversation with self' and is enhanced by reflective discussions with another person. It demonstrates *par excellence* the process of continuing professional development and provides a means of displaying this to another person, and the use of qualitative assessment approaches that are open and capable of being validated allows judgements to be made about the writer.

A portfolio approach has the potential to encourage, capture and record deep approaches to learning, through an active search for meaning, personal significance and linking to existing knowledge. Portfolios provide the opportunity for a reflective approach that allows experiences to be replayed and critically reconstructed in a way that identifies and highlights educational needs and thereby points the way for future learning. The philosophy is learner centred; the learner takes responsibility for planning and demonstrating that learning has occurred. While initially the approach is often negatively influenced by attitudes related to uncertainty and unfamiliarity, it is clear that for many writers, portfolios can become an acceptable and often welcome form of recording continuing professional development and an assessment method which is seen as fair and transparent. Maintaining a portfolio throughout a career is a powerful means of demonstrating commitment, continued learning and career development.

It is likely that from a purely psychometric viewpoint, criticisms can be made of any existing method of portfolio assessment. The essentially subjective nature of a reflective portfolio represents a technical rationalist's nightmare, and their response might be to enforce such a degree of standardisation that reflective learning would be lost in the need to meet some standard of performance. However, from the professional artistry perspective, a portfolio has the potential to demonstrate the very essence of professionalism: capturing reflection, deliberation, insights and creativity. This requires some changes to our traditional ways of thinking.

Acknowledgement

Some of the material used in this paper has previously been published in two articles by the author [93,94] in *Medical Teacher* and is reproduced here with permission.

References

1 Royal College of General Practitioners (1993) *Portfolio Based Learning in General Practice*. Royal College of General Practitioners, London.

2 Redman W (1994) *Portfolios for Development; a guide for trainers and managers*. Kogan - Page, London.

3 Flanagan J (1954) The critical incident technique. *Psychological Bulletin*. **51**: 327–58.

4 Pringle M, Bradley C, Carmichael C, Wallis H and Moore A (1997) *Significant Event Auditing*. Royal College of General Practitioners, London.

5 Rees C (2005) The use (and abuse) of the term 'portfolio'. *Medical Education*. **39**: 436.

6 Paulson F, Paulson P and Meyer C (1991) What makes a portfolio a portfolio? *Educational Leadership*. **48**: 60–3.

7 Brown R (1992) *Portfolio Development and Profiling for Nurses*. Quay Publishing, Lancaster.

8 Hall D (1992) Professional development portfolios for teachers and lecturers. *British Journal of In-service Education*. **18**: 81–6.

9 Webb C (2002) Models of portfolios. *Medical Education*. **36**: 897–8.

10 Parboosingh J and McLaughlin R (1996) Learning portfolios: potential to assist health professionals with self directed learning. *Journal of Continuing Education in the Health Professions*. **16**: 75–81.

11 Fung M, Walker M, Fung K, Temple L, Lajoie F, Bellemare G and Bryson S (2000) An internet-based learning portfolio in resident education: the KOALA multicentre programme. *Medical Education*. **34**: 474–9.

12 NHS Education Scotland (2006) *Foundation Programme Portfolio* (www.nhsdots.org/nhsdots/dotsx/login.asp; last accessed 10 October 2006).

13 NHS (2006) *Appraisal Toolkit* (www.apraisals.nhs.uk; last accessed 10 October 2006).

14 Dagley V and Berrington B (2005) Learning from an evaluation of an electronic portfolio to support general practitioners' personal development, planning, appraisal and revalidation. *Education for Primary Care*. **16**: 567–74.

15 Davis M, Ben-David M, Harden R, Howie P, Ker JmcGhee C, Pippard M and Snadden D (2001) Portfolio assessment in medical students' final examinations. *Medical Teacher*. **23**: 357–66.

16 Tomkinson B (1997) *Towards a Taxonomy of Teaching Portfolios*. University of Manchester, Manchester.

17 Friedman S and Marr J (1995) A supervisory model of professional competence: a joint service/education initiative. *Nurse Education Today*. **15**: 239–44.

18 Melland H and Volden C (1996) Teaching portfolios for faculty evaluation. *Nurse Educator*. **21**: 35–8.

19 Oermann N (1999) Developing a teaching portfolio. *Journal of Professional Nursing.* **15**: 224–8.

20 Treasure W (1996) Portfolio-based learning pilot scheme for general practitioner principals in south-east Scotland. *Education for General Practice.* **7**: 249–54.

21 Pitts J and Vincent S (1995) A higher professional education course in Wessex – the first year. *Education for General Practice.* **6**: 157–62.

22 Snadden D, Thomas M, Griffin E and Hudson H (1996) Portfolio-based learning and general practice vocational training. *Medical Education.* **30**: 148–52.

23 Snadden D and Thomas M (1998) The use of portfolio learning in medical education. *Medical Teacher.* **20**: 192–9.

24 Challis M, Mathers N, Howe A and Field N (1997) Portfolio-based learning: continuing medical education for general practitioners – a mid-point evaluation. *Medical Education.* **31**: 22–6.

25 Calman K (1998) *A Review of Continuing Professional Development in Practice: a report to the Secretary of State from the Chief Medical Officer.* Department of Health, London.

26 Pitts J, Curtis A, While R and Holloway I (1999) 'Practice Professional Development Plans': general practitioners' perspectives on proposed changes in general practice education. *British Journal of General Practice.* **49**: 959–62.

27 Brigley S (2001) *Y Portffolio: the development of portfolio learning among groups of general practitioners in Wales.* University of Wales College of Medicine, Cardiff.

28 Dornan T, Carroll C and Parboosingh J (2002) An electronic learning portfolio for reflective continuing professional development. *Medical Education.* **36**: 767–9.

29 Jasper M (1995) The potential of the professional portfolio for nursing. *Journal of Clinical Nursing.* **4**: 249–55.

30 O'Mara L, Carpio B, Mallete C, Down W and Brown B (2000) Developing a teaching portfolio in nursing education: a reflection. *Nurse Educator.* **25**: 125–9.

31 Cayne J (1995) Portfolios as a developmental influence. *Journal of Advanced Nursing.* **21**: 395–405.

32 Grant J, Ramsey A and Bain J (1997) Community hospitals and general practice: extended attachments for students. *Medical Education.* **31**: 364–8.

33 Driessen E, Tartwijk J, Vermunt J and van der Vleuten C (2003) Use of portfolios in early undergraduate medical education. *Medical Teacher.* **25**: 18–23.

34 Beecher A, Lindemann J, Morzinski J and Simpson D (1997) Use of the educator's portfolio to stimulate reflective practice among medical educators. *Teaching and Learning in Medicine.* **9**: 56–9.

35 Kelly D and Murray T (1999) The development and evaluation of a personal learning log for senior house officers. *Medical Education.* **33**: 260–6.

36 Campbell C, Parboosingh J, Gondocz T, Babitskaya G and Pham B (1996) Study of the factors influencing the stimulus to learning recorded by physicians keeping a learning portfolio. *Journal of Continuing Education in the Health Professions.* **19**: 16–24.

37 Tigelaar D, Dolmans D, de Grave W, Wolfhagen I and van der Vleuten C (2006) Portfolio as a tool to stimulate teachers reflections. *Medical Teacher.* **28**: 277–82.

38 Tigelaar D, Dolmans D, de Grave W, Wolfhagen I and van der Vleuten C (2006) Participants' opinions on the usefulness of a teaching portfolio. *Medical Education.* **40**: 371–8.

39 Lonka K, Slotte V, Halttunen M, Kurki T, Tiitinen A, Vaara L and Paavonen J (2001) Portfolios as a learning tool in obstetrics and gynaecology undergraduate training. *Medical Education.* **35**: 1125–30.

40 General Medical Council (1997) *The New Doctor.* GMC, London.

41 Department of Health (1998) *A Guide to Specialist Registrar Training.* Department of Health, London.

42 Pitts J, Coles C and Thomas P (1999) Educational portfolios in the assessment of general practice trainers: reliability of assessors. *Medical Education.* **33**: 515–20.

43 Roberts C (2002) Portfolio-based assessments in medical education: are they valid and reliable for summative purposes? *Medical Education.* **36**: 899–900.

44 Gordon MJ (1991) A review of the validity and accuracy of self-assessments in health professions training. *Academic Medicine.* **66**: 762–9.

45 McKinstry B and Evans A (2006) Self-assessment or self-delusion? *Education for Primary Care.* **17**: 432–5.

46 Rees C and Sheard C (2004) The reliability of assessment criteria for undergraduate medical students' communication skills portfolios; the Nottingham experience. *Medical Education.* **38**: 138–44.

47 Roberts C, Cromarty I, Crossley J and Jolly B (2006) The reliability and validity of a matrix to assess the completed reflective personal development plans of general practitioners. *Medical Education.* **40**: 363–70.

48 Driessen E, van Tartwijk J, Overeem K, Vermunt J and van der Vleuten C (2005) Conditions for successful reflective use of portfolios in undergraduate medical education. *Medical Education.* **39**: 214–20.

49 Karlowicz K (2000) The value of student portfolios to evaluate undergraduate nursing programmes. *Nurse Educator.* **25**: 82–7.

50 Speer A and Elnicki D (1999) Assessing the quality of teaching. *American Journal of Medicine.* **106**: 381–3.

51 Lee L, Froh R and Petrusa E (1997) Assessing the implementation of teaching portfolios in the academic medical center. In: Scherpbier A *et al*. (eds) *Advances in Medical Education*. Kluwer Academic Publishers, Dordrecht.

52 Murray E, Alderman P, Coppola W, Grol R, Bouhuijs P and van der Vleuten C (2001) What do students actually do on an internal medicine clerkship? A log diary study. *Medical Education*. **35**: 1101–7.

53 United Kingdom Central Council for Nursing (1994) *The Future of Professional Practice. The Council's Standard for Education and Practice Following Registration*. UKCC, London.

54 English National Board (1991) *Professional Portfolio*. ENB, London.

55 Jasper M (1995) The portfolio workbook as a strategy for student-centred learning. *Nurse Education Today*. **15**: 446–51.

56 General Medical Council (2001) *Good Medical Practice*. GMC, London.

57 Deckert B (1990) Reach for excellence – a clinical ladder promotion system. *Journal of the American Nursing Association*. **17**: 296–8.

58 Oechsle L, Volden C and Lambeth S (1990) Portfolios and RNs; an evaluation. *Journal of Nursing Education*. **29**: 54–9.

59 Simpson D, Morzinski J, Beecher A and Lindemann J (1994) Meeting the challenge to document teaching accomplishments: the educator's portfolio. *Teaching and Learning in Medicine*. **6**: 203–6.

60 Beasley B, Wright S, Cofrancesco J, Babbott S, Thomas P and Bass E (1997) Promotion criteria for clinician educators in the United States and Canada. *Journal of the American Medical Association*. **278**: 723–8.

61 Niemi P (1997) Medical students' professional identity: self-reflection during the pre-clinical years. *Medical Education*. **31**: 408–15.

62 Al-Shehri A (1995) Learning by reflection in general practice: a study report. *Education for General Practice*. **7**: 237–48.

63 Newmann F (1990) Higher order thinking in teaching social studies: a rationale for the assessment of classroom thoughtfulness. *Journal of Curriculum Studies*. **22**: 41–56.

64 Schuwirth L and van der Vleuten C (2006) A plea for new psychometric models in educational assessment. *Medical Education*. **40**: 296–300.

65 Pitts J and Coles C (2003) The challenge of non-standardised assessment of professionals – the need for a paradigm shift. *Education for Primary Care*. **14**: 397–405.

66 Moss P (1994) Can there be validity without reliability? *Educational Researcher*. **23**: 5–12.

67 Davis M and Fleiss J (1982) Measuring agreement for multinomial data. *Biometrics*. **38**: 1047–51.

68 Newble D and Jaeger K (1983) The effects of assessments and examinations on the learning of medical students. *Medical Education*. **17**: 165–71.

69 Phillips D (1990) Subjectivity and objectivity: an objective enquiry. In: Eisner E and Peshkin A (eds) *Qualitative Enquiry in Education – the continuing debate*. Teachers College Press, New York.

70 Pitts J, Coles C, Thomas P and Smith F (2002) Enhancing reliability in portfolio assessment: discussions between assessors. *Medical Teacher.* **24**: 197–201.

71 Van der Vleuten C (1996) The assessment of professional competence: developments, research and practical implications. *Advances in Health Sciences Education.* **1**: 41–67.

72 Dewey J (1933) *How We Think: a restatement of the relation between reflective thinking to the educative process*. DC Heath, London.

73 Schön D (1983) *The Reflective Practitioner.* Jossey-Bass, San Francisco, CA.

74 Boyd E and Fales A (1983) Reflective learning: key to learning from experience. *Journal of Humanistic Psychology.* **23**: 99–117.

75 Schön D (1987) *Educating the Reflective Practitioner.* Jossey-Bass, San Francisco, CA.

76 Bines H and Watson D (1992) *Developing Professional Education*. Open University Press, Milton Keynes.

77 Boud D and Walker D (1993) Barriers to reflection on experience. In: Boud D, Cohen R and Walker D (eds) *Using Experience for Learning*. Open University Press, Milton Keynes.

78 Kolb D and Fry R (1975) Towards an applied theory of experiential learning. In: Cooper C (ed.) *Theories of Group Practices*. John Wiley and Sons, London.

79 Jarvis P (1987) *Adult Learning in the Social Context.* Croom Helm, London.

80 Sparks-Langer G and Colton A (1991) Synthesis of research on teachers' reflective learning. *Educational Leadership.* **48**: 37–44.

81 Ross D (1990) Programmatic structures for the preparation of reflective teachers. In: Clift R, Houston W and Pugach M (eds) *Encouraging Reflective Practice in Education*. Teachers College Press, New York.

82 Lave J and Wenger E (1991) *Situated Learning: legitimate peripheral participation*. Cambridge University Press, Cambridge.

83 Hanks W (1991) Foreword. In: Lave J and Wenger E. *Situated Learning: legitimate peripheral participation*. Cambridge University Press, Cambridge.

84 Wenzel L, Briggs K and Puryear B (1998) Portfolio: authentic assessment in the age of the curriculum revolution. *Journal of Nursing Education.* **37**: 208–12.

85 Eraut M (1994) *Developing Professional Knowledge and Competence.* Falmer Press, London.

86 Coles C (2000) *Credentialing Through the Natural Processes of Continuing Professional Development: what more do we need?* American Board of Medical Specialties, Chicago.

87 Fish D (1991) But can you prove it? Quality assurance and the reflective practitioner. *Assessment and Evaluation in Higher Education.* **16**: 22–36.

88 Passmore J (1989) *The Philosophy of Teaching.* Duckworth Press, London.

89 Simosko S (1991) *APL: a practical guide for professionals.* Kogan-Page, London.

90 Woodward H (1998) Reflective journals and portfolios: learning through assessment. *Assessment and Evaluation in Higher Education.* **23**: 415–23.

91 Solomon P (1992) Learning contracts in clinical education: evaluation by clinical supervisors. *Medical Teacher.* **14**: 205–10.

92 Martenson D and Schwab P (1993) Learning through mutual commitment: broadening the concept of learning contracts. *Medical Teacher.* **15**: 11–15.

93 Pitts J, Coles C and Thomas P (2001) Enhancing reliability in portfolio assessment: shaping the portfolio. *Medical Teacher.* **23**: 351–6.

94 Pitts J, Coles C, Thomas P and Smith F (2002) Enhancing reliability in portfolio assessment: discussion between assessors. *Medical Teacher.* **24**: 197–201.

Further reading

Ben-David M, Davis M, Harden R, Howie P, Ker J and Pippard M (2001) AMEE Medical Education Guide No. 24: portfolios as a method of student assessment. *Medical Teacher.* **23**: 535–51.

Challis M (1999) AMEE Medical Education Guide No. 11: portfolio-based learning and assessment in medical education. *Medical Teacher.* **22**: 370–86.

Klenowski V (2002) *Developing Portfolios for Learning and Assessment. Processes and Principles.* London: Routledge-Falmer.

About ASME

The Association for the Study of Medical Education (ASME) seeks to improve the quality of medical education by bringing together individuals and organisations with interests and responsibilities in medical and healthcare education.

ASME is unique in that it draws its members from all areas of medical education – undergraduate, postgraduate and continuing – and from all specialties. It has a function as a forum for debate and exchange of information, and is building on its contacts in medicine and teaching in the UK and among other networks, to promote knowledge and expertise in medical education.

ASME seeks to:

- promote high-quality research into medical education
- provide opportunities for developing medical educators
- disseminate good evidence-based educational practice
- inform and advise governmental and other organisations on medical education matters
- develop relationships with other organisations and groupings in healthcare education.

ASME's values are:

- education and learning are central to the delivery of high-quality healthcare
- education must be an important component in the strategies of governmental and other healthcare organisations
- good healthcare educators are central in planning, delivering and evaluating high-quality healthcare
- individual members of ASME should be supported and developed
- high-quality research is necessary for the development of healthcare education
- vision, innovation and leadership in healthcare education are to be fostered.